Awesome Beginners Guide to Healthy Living for Men

The Importance of Wellness Strategies for Men

By

Beathan Clark

Copyright@2023

Table of Contents

CHAPTER 1

Introduction

1.1 What is Men's Health?

Men's health is a multidimensional concept encompassing physical, mental, and social well-being that is specific to the male population. It focuses on addressing the unique health needs and challenges that men face throughout their lives. This field of health and medicine recognizes that men, like women, have their own set of health concerns that require attention, education, and proactive management.

Men's health covers a wide range of issues, including but not limited to:

1. **Physical Health**: This involves the prevention, diagnosis, and treatment of medical conditions that primarily affect men. These conditions can range from heart disease, prostate cancer, and erectile dysfunction to issues related to fitness, nutrition, and sexual health.

2. **Mental Health**: Men's mental health is an essential aspect of overall well-being. It encompasses emotional and psychological health, addressing issues such as depression, anxiety, stress, and the stigma often associated with seeking help for mental health challenges.

3. **Social Health**: Social health involves the quality of relationships and social

connections in a man's life. This can include family relationships, friendships, and community involvement. Maintaining strong social ties is vital for emotional support and overall happiness.

4. **Behavioral Health**: This aspect of men's health addresses lifestyle choices and behaviors that impact health. It includes areas such as smoking, alcohol consumption, substance abuse, and risky behaviors, emphasizing the importance of making healthier choices.

5. **Preventive Care**: Men's health emphasizes the significance of preventive measures, such as regular health check-ups and screenings, to catch and address potential health issues early,

before they become more serious.

6. **Healthy Aging**: As men age, their health needs change. Men's health includes guidance on navigating the aging process, addressing age-related concerns, and maintaining a high quality of life as they grow older.

1.2 The Importance of Men's Health

The importance of men's health cannot be overstated, as it directly affects not only individual men but also their families, communities, and society as a whole. Here are several key reasons why men's health is of paramount importance:

1. **Reducing Mortality**: Men have a higher mortality rate than women for many common health conditions, including heart disease, cancer, and accidents. Focusing on men's health can help reduce premature deaths and improve overall life expectancy.

2. **Enhancing Quality of Life**: Good health is a foundation for a fulfilling life. By addressing men's unique health concerns, we can enhance their physical and mental well-being, leading to happier, more productive lives.

3. **Preventing Chronic Diseases**: Many chronic diseases, such as diabetes and hypertension, can often be prevented or managed effectively with early

intervention and lifestyle modifications. Regular health check-ups and healthy habits can play a crucial role in preventing these conditions.

4. **Promoting Family Health**: Men's health is closely tied to family health. When men take care of themselves, they are better able to support their families, both emotionally and financially.

5. **Reducing Healthcare Costs**: Preventive care and early intervention are cost-effective approaches to healthcare. By promoting men's health and preventing chronic conditions, we can reduce the economic burden of healthcare on individuals and society.

6. **Mental Health and Well-being**: Addressing men's mental health is vital in reducing the stigma associated with seeking help for mental health issues. It can lead to improved emotional resilience, healthier relationships, and a better overall quality of life.

men's health is a multifaceted concept that encompasses physical, mental, and social well-being specific to men. Recognizing and prioritizing men's health is essential for improving individual lives, reducing mortality, and building healthier communities and societies. It requires a proactive approach to healthcare, preventive measures, and a commitment to addressing the unique health challenges that men face at different stages of life.

1.3 Common Health Concerns for Men

Men, like women, have specific health concerns that they should be aware of and actively manage throughout their lives. These concerns can vary depending on factors such as age, genetics, lifestyle, and overall health status. Here are some of the common health concerns that men should pay attention to:

1. Cardiovascular Disease:

- Heart disease is a leading cause of death in men. Risk factors include high blood pressure, high cholesterol, smoking, obesity, and a family history of heart disease. Regular exercise, a heart-healthy diet, and stress management are essential for heart health.

2. Prostate Health:

- Prostate problems, including benign prostatic hyperplasia (enlarged prostate) and prostate cancer, are common as men age. Regular prostate screenings and discussions with healthcare providers are crucial for early detection and treatment.

3. Testicular Health:

- Testicular cancer is the most common cancer among young men. Men should perform regular testicular self-exams and report any unusual lumps, pain, or changes to their healthcare providers.

4. Sexual Health:

- Sexual health concerns, such as erectile dysfunction, low testosterone levels, and sexually transmitted infections (STIs), can affect a man's overall well-being. Open communication with a healthcare provider is essential for addressing these issues.

5. Mental Health:

- Men may be less likely to seek help for mental health problems, but conditions like depression and anxiety can have a significant impact on their lives. Recognizing the signs, seeking support, and addressing mental health challenges is crucial.

6. Obesity and Weight Management:

- Obesity is associated with various health issues, including diabetes, heart disease, and joint problems. Maintaining a healthy weight through diet and exercise is essential for preventing these conditions.

7. Diabetes:

- Men are at risk for both type 1 and type 2 diabetes. Regular blood glucose monitoring and lifestyle modifications, including a balanced diet and physical activity, are vital for diabetes prevention and management.

8. Hypertension (High Blood Pressure):

- High blood pressure can lead to heart disease, stroke, and other health problems. Monitoring blood pressure regularly and following treatment plans if diagnosed is crucial.

9. Lung Health:

- Smoking is a major risk factor for lung cancer and respiratory diseases. Quitting smoking and avoiding exposure to environmental toxins is essential for lung health.

10. Osteoporosis: - Although less common in men, osteoporosis can occur and lead to fragile bones and fractures. Adequate calcium intake, vitamin D, and weight-bearing exercise can help maintain bone health.

11. Substance Abuse and Addiction: - Men are more likely to engage in risky behaviors involving alcohol and drugs. Substance abuse can have severe physical, mental, and social consequences and should be addressed through treatment and support.

12. Accidents and Injuries: - Men are more prone to accidents and injuries, often due to risk-taking behaviors. Practicing safety measures and using protective equipment can reduce the risk of accidents.

13. Aging-Related Concerns: - As men age, they may face age-related issues such as decreased muscle mass, cognitive decline, and an increased risk of certain health conditions. Regular healthcare check-ups and a focus on healthy aging strategies are important.

It's crucial for men to be proactive about their health by scheduling regular check-ups, adopting a healthy lifestyle, and seeking medical advice when needed. Early detection and prevention are key to managing and mitigating many of these common health concerns.

CHAPTER 2

Preventive Measures

Preventive measures play a pivotal role in maintaining good health and reducing the risk of various health conditions. In the context of men's health, these measures encompass regular health check-ups, adopting healthy lifestyle choices, and paying attention to nutrition and diet.

2.1 Regular Health Check-ups

Regular health check-ups are essential for monitoring your overall health, detecting potential issues early, and maintaining a proactive approach to wellness. Here's why they are crucial:

- **Early Detection:** Regular check-ups can help identify health problems in their early stages, when they are often more manageable and treatable.

- **Screening Tests:** These exams may include blood pressure measurement, cholesterol level checks, blood glucose tests, and screenings for specific conditions like prostate cancer or colorectal cancer.

- **Health Monitoring:** Check-ups provide an opportunity to track your weight, blood pressure, and other vital signs over time, allowing healthcare providers to assess your health trends.

- **Vaccinations:** Immunizations, such as flu shots and vaccines for preventable diseases, are typically discussed and administered during check-ups.

- **Preventive Counseling:** Healthcare providers can offer guidance on lifestyle changes, such as smoking cessation, weight management, and stress reduction.

- **Personalized Care:** Regular visits allow you to build a relationship with your healthcare provider, enabling them to tailor their advice and recommendations to your specific health needs.

- **Medication Management:** If you have an existing medical condition, check-ups ensure that your medications are working effectively and that any necessary adjustments are made.

It's recommended that men schedule regular check-ups with their primary care physician or healthcare provider, with the frequency of these visits varying based on age, existing health conditions, and individual risk factors.

2.2 Healthy Lifestyle Choices

Healthy lifestyle choices have a profound impact on overall health and can significantly reduce the risk of chronic diseases. Here are key aspects of adopting a healthy lifestyle:

- **Physical Activity:** Regular exercise, such as aerobic activities, strength training, and flexibility exercises, helps

maintain a healthy weight,
improve cardiovascular health,
and boost overall well-being.

- **Balanced Diet:** A diet rich in
  fruits, vegetables, whole grains,
  lean proteins, and healthy fats
  provides essential nutrients and
  reduces the risk of obesity,
  heart disease, and diabetes.

- **Tobacco and Alcohol Use:**
  Quitting smoking and
  moderating alcohol
  consumption are critical for
  reducing the risk of lung
  cancer, cardiovascular disease,
  and liver problems.

- **Stress Management:**
  Techniques like mindfulness,
  meditation, and relaxation
  exercises can help manage

stress, which is linked to various health issues.

- **Adequate Sleep:** Getting sufficient sleep is essential for mental and physical health, as it supports cognitive function, immune function, and overall well-being.

- **Limiting Risky Behaviors:** Avoiding risky behaviors such as reckless driving and substance abuse reduces the risk of accidents and injuries.

- **Regular Health Screenings:** Adhering to recommended screenings for conditions like diabetes, hypertension, and cancer is an integral part of a healthy lifestyle.

2.3 Nutrition and Diet

Nutrition and diet play a central role in men's health. A well-balanced diet provides the body with essential nutrients and energy while reducing the risk of chronic diseases. Consider the following dietary principles:

- **Fruits and Vegetables:** Aim to consume a variety of colorful fruits and vegetables daily, as they are rich in vitamins, minerals, fiber, and antioxidants that promote health and reduce the risk of chronic diseases.

- **Whole Grains:** Opt for whole grains like brown rice, whole wheat bread, and oats instead of refined grains to increase fiber intake and support digestive health.

- **Lean Protein:** Include sources of lean protein such as poultry, fish, beans, tofu, and legumes in your diet. Protein is essential for muscle health and overall body function.

- **Healthy Fats:** Choose sources of healthy fats like avocados, nuts, seeds, and olive oil while limiting saturated and trans fats found in fried and processed foods.

- **Portion Control:** Pay attention to portion sizes to avoid overeating, which can lead to weight gain and related health issues.

- **Hydration:** Drink plenty of water throughout the day to stay well-hydrated and support various bodily functions.

- **Limit Added Sugars and Sodium:** Reduce the consumption of foods and beverages high in added sugars and sodium, as they can contribute to health problems such as obesity and high blood pressure.

- **Moderate Alcohol Consumption:** If you choose to consume alcohol, do so in moderation, following recommended guidelines to minimize health risks.

A registered dietitian or nutritionist can provide personalized dietary recommendations based on your health goals and needs. By incorporating these healthy lifestyle choices and focusing on nutrition, men can take proactive steps to maintain their health and well-being.

2.4 Exercise and Physical Activity

Exercise and physical activity are fundamental components of a healthy lifestyle and are critical for men's health. Regular exercise provides numerous physical and mental health benefits. Here's a closer look at why exercise is essential and how to incorporate it into your life:

Physical Health Benefits:

1. **Weight Management:** Regular exercise helps control body weight by burning calories and increasing metabolism, reducing the risk of obesity-related conditions.

2. **Heart Health:** Exercise strengthens the heart, lowers blood pressure, and improves

cholesterol levels, reducing the risk of heart disease and stroke.

3. **Muscle and Bone Health:** Weight-bearing exercises, such as strength training, help build and maintain muscle mass and bone density, reducing the risk of osteoporosis.

4. **Diabetes Prevention:** Physical activity improves insulin sensitivity and helps prevent or manage type 2 diabetes.

5. **Cancer Risk Reduction:** Exercise may lower the risk of certain cancers, including colon and breast cancer.

Mental Health Benefits:

1. **Stress Reduction:** Physical activity releases endorphins, which are natural mood lifters,

helping to reduce stress and improve overall well-being.

2. **Anxiety and Depression Management:** Regular exercise can be an effective tool in managing symptoms of anxiety and depression by promoting relaxation and improving self-esteem.

3. **Enhanced Cognitive Function:** Exercise has cognitive benefits, including improved memory, attention, and problem-solving skills.

4. **Better Sleep:** Regular physical activity can improve sleep quality and help with insomnia.

Tips for Incorporating Exercise:

- Find activities you enjoy, whether it's running, cycling,

swimming, team sports, or dancing, to make exercise more enjoyable and sustainable.

- Aim for at least 150 minutes of moderate-intensity aerobic exercise or 75 minutes of vigorous-intensity aerobic exercise per week, along with muscle-strengthening activities on two or more days a week.

- Start slowly if you're new to exercise and gradually increase the duration and intensity of your workouts to prevent injuries.

- Make exercise a part of your daily routine by scheduling it like an appointment.

- Consider seeking guidance from a fitness professional or personal trainer to develop a safe and effective exercise program tailored to your goals and fitness level.

2.5 Mental Health and Stress Management

Mental health and stress management are integral components of men's overall well-being. Paying attention to your mental health is crucial for maintaining a healthy and balanced life. Here's why mental health and stress management are vital and how to prioritize them:

Mental Health Importance:

1. **Emotional Well-being:** Good mental health supports emotional stability, helping individuals cope with life's challenges and setbacks.

2. **Relationships:** Healthy mental health enhances relationships by promoting effective communication and emotional intimacy.

3. **Productivity:** Mental well-being is linked to increased productivity and job satisfaction.

4. **Quality of Life:** A positive mental outlook contributes to an improved quality of life, greater life satisfaction, and happiness.

Stress Management:

1. **Identify Stressors:** Recognize the sources of stress in your life, whether they are work-related, personal, or environmental.

2. **Practice Relaxation Techniques:** Incorporate relaxation methods like deep breathing, meditation, and progressive muscle relaxation into your daily routine to reduce stress.

3. **Physical Activity:** Regular exercise, as mentioned earlier, is an effective stress reliever.

4. **Time Management:** Prioritize tasks, set realistic goals, and manage your time effectively to reduce feelings of overwhelm.

5. **Social Support:** Maintain a support system of friends and family with whom you can share your feelings and concerns.

6. **Seek Professional Help:** If stress becomes overwhelming

or leads to persistent anxiety or depression, consider seeking help from a mental health professional.

7. **Healthy Lifestyle:** Nutrition, exercise, and sleep play a role in stress management. A balanced lifestyle can better equip you to cope with stress.

8. **Limit Stressors:** When possible, take steps to reduce or eliminate sources of chronic stress in your life, whether it's through job changes, adjusting your routine, or seeking help with financial challenges.

Taking care of your mental health is not a sign of weakness but a sign of strength and self-awareness. Prioritizing mental health and effective stress management can lead to improved overall health and a higher quality of life.

CHAPTER 3

Common Men's Health Issues

Common men's health issues encompass a range of conditions and concerns that affect men's physical and emotional well-being. In this section, we'll explore three significant areas: heart health, prostate health, and sexual health.

3.1 Heart Health

Heart health is a critical aspect of men's overall well-being, as heart disease remains one of the leading causes of death for men worldwide.

Key points regarding heart health for men include:

- **Risk Factors:** Men are more prone to certain risk factors, including high blood pressure, high cholesterol, obesity, and smoking, which increase the likelihood of heart disease.

- **Prevention:** Adopting a heart-healthy lifestyle can significantly reduce the risk of heart disease. This includes maintaining a balanced diet, engaging in regular physical activity, quitting smoking, and managing stress.

- **Symptoms:** Men should be aware of heart attack symptoms, which can include chest pain or discomfort, shortness of breath, fatigue, and pain in the arm, neck, jaw, or back. Recognizing these signs and seeking immediate medical attention is crucial.

- **Screening:** Regular blood pressure and cholesterol checks, along with discussions about heart health with a healthcare provider, are essential for early detection and management of cardiovascular risk factors.

3.2 Prostate Health

Prostate health is a specific concern for men, with conditions such as benign prostatic hyperplasia (BPH) and prostate cancer being of particular importance:

- **Benign Prostatic Hyperplasia (BPH):** BPH is a common condition in older men characterized by an enlarged prostate gland. Symptoms can include urinary frequency, urgency, and difficulty starting or stopping urination. Treatment options range from medication to surgical procedures.

- **Prostate Cancer:** Prostate cancer is one of the most common cancers in men. Early detection is crucial for successful treatment. Regular prostate-specific antigen (PSA) tests and discussions with healthcare providers are essential for monitoring prostate health.

3.3 Sexual Health

Sexual health encompasses a wide range of physical and psychological aspects of a man's sexual well-being:

- **Erectile Dysfunction (ED):** ED is a common condition that can affect men of all ages. It involves difficulty achieving or maintaining an erection sufficient for sexual intercourse. Various treatment options, including medication, lifestyle changes, and counseling, can help manage ED.

- **Low Testosterone:** Some men experience low testosterone levels, which can lead to symptoms such as fatigue, reduced libido, and mood changes. Hormone replacement therapy may be considered in consultation with a healthcare provider.

- **Sexually Transmitted Infections (STIs):** Practicing safe sex and using protection, such as condoms, is essential to prevent STIs. Regular STI screenings are advisable, especially if you are sexually active with multiple partners.

- **Fertility:** Fertility concerns may arise for men experiencing difficulties with reproduction. A thorough evaluation by a specialist can help identify potential causes and treatment options.

- **Mental Health and Intimacy:** Psychological factors, such as stress, anxiety, and depression, can affect sexual health. Open communication with a partner and, if needed, mental health support or counseling can help address these issues.

Men's sexual health is a vital component of their overall well-being and should not be overlooked. It is essential to seek medical advice and support when facing sexual health challenges, as they can often be effectively managed or treated with the appropriate interventions.

3.4 Testicular Health

Testicular health is a critical aspect of men's well-being, and understanding how to maintain it and detect potential issues is essential. Here's an overview of testicular health:

- **Testicular Self-Exams:**
Regular testicular self-exams
are a valuable practice for men
to detect potential abnormalities
early. During self-exams, men
can feel for lumps, changes in
size, or other irregularities in
their testicles. Any concerning
findings should be promptly
discussed with a healthcare
provider.

- **Testicular Cancer:** Testicular
cancer is relatively rare but is
the most common cancer
among young men. It typically
occurs in men aged 15 to 44.
Early detection and treatment
can result in high survival rates.
Signs of testicular cancer may
include pain or discomfort,
swelling, or a lump in the
testicles.

- **Risk Factors:** While the exact cause of testicular cancer is not known, certain risk factors, such as a family history of the disease and prior testicular cancer, may increase the likelihood. Understanding these risk factors can help men make informed decisions about their health.

- **Treatment:** Testicular cancer is highly treatable, often with surgery to remove the affected testicle. Depending on the stage and type of cancer, additional treatments such as radiation therapy or chemotherapy may be necessary.

3.5 Mental Health and Depression

Mental health is a vital aspect of overall well-being, and men should be aware of the importance of mental health and how to address issues such as depression:

- **Prevalence of Depression:** Depression is a common mental health condition that can affect men of all ages. It often presents differently in men, with symptoms like irritability, anger, and physical complaints sometimes being more prominent than sadness.

- **Seeking Help:** Men may be less likely to seek help for mental health concerns due to stigma or a perception of weakness. It's essential to recognize the signs of depression, such as persistent sadness, loss of interest in activities, changes in appetite or sleep, and fatigue, and to seek professional support when needed.

- **Treatment:** Depression is treatable with various approaches, including therapy, medication, lifestyle changes, and support from loved ones. Effective treatment can lead to symptom relief and improved quality of life.

- **Preventive Measures:** Mental health promotion involves stress management, self-care, seeking social support, and adopting a healthy lifestyle, all of which can help prevent or mitigate the risk of depression.

3.6 Substance Abuse and Addiction

Substance abuse and addiction are significant concerns for men's health, as they can have severe physical, mental, and social consequences:

- **Substance Abuse:** Substance abuse involves the harmful or hazardous use of substances like alcohol, tobacco, prescription drugs, or illicit drugs. It can lead to health problems, impaired judgment, accidents, and strained relationships.

- **Addiction:** Addiction is characterized by a physical or psychological dependence on a substance. Overcoming addiction often requires specialized treatment and support to achieve and maintain recovery.

- **Mental Health Connection:** Substance abuse and addiction are often linked to mental health issues, such as depression, anxiety, and trauma. Addressing both the substance use disorder and co-occurring mental health conditions is essential for successful recovery.

- **Treatment Options:** Treatment for substance abuse and addiction may include detoxification, counseling, behavioral therapy, medication-assisted treatment, and support groups. It's crucial for individuals struggling with addiction to seek help from professionals and support networks.

- **Prevention:** Prevention efforts focus on educating individuals about the risks of substance abuse, promoting healthy coping mechanisms, and providing resources for early intervention.

Understanding the importance of testicular health, mental health, and the risks associated with substance abuse and addiction is essential for men's overall well-being. Early detection and seeking appropriate support and treatment for any of these issues are crucial steps toward maintaining a healthy and fulfilling life.

CHAPTER 4

Age-Related Health Concerns

Men's health needs and concerns evolve throughout their lifespan, with distinct health considerations during adolescence, adulthood, and the senior years. Here's an overview of age-related health concerns for men at each stage:

4.1 Men's Health in Adolescence

Adolescence is a critical period of growth and development, and it sets the foundation for a man's health in adulthood. Key health considerations during adolescence include:

- **Physical Growth:** Adolescents experience significant physical growth, including the development of secondary sexual characteristics, such as facial hair and muscle mass. Proper nutrition and exercise are crucial for healthy growth.

- **Sexual Health Education:** Adolescents should receive comprehensive sexual health education, including information about safe sex practices, sexually transmitted infections (STIs), and contraception.

- **Mental Health:** Adolescence can be a challenging time, with emotional and psychological changes. Promoting good mental health, coping skills, and self-esteem is essential.

- **Substance Use Prevention:** Adolescents may experiment with drugs, alcohol, or tobacco. Prevention programs and open communication about the risks of substance abuse are crucial.

- **Physical Activity:** Encouraging physical activity and the development of healthy exercise habits is essential for long-term health.

4.2 Men's Health in Adulthood

Adulthood encompasses a wide range of ages, from the late teens to midlife and beyond. Health concerns evolve during this period:

- **Heart Health:** Cardiovascular health becomes increasingly

important, with factors like
diet, exercise, and stress
management playing a
significant role in preventing
heart disease.

- **Prostate Health:** Screening for
prostate cancer typically begins
in adulthood, with regular
discussions about prostate
health and potential concerns.

- **Mental Health:** The pressures
of work, family, and financial
responsibilities can impact
mental health. Seeking support
for stress, anxiety, and
depression is critical.

- **Reproductive Health:** Men
may consider family planning,
and discussions about fertility
and contraception may become
relevant.

- **Bone Health:** Bone density and muscle mass may start to decline, making it important to maintain regular exercise and adequate nutrition.

4.3 Men's Health in the Senior Years

As men enter their senior years, additional health considerations come into play:

- **Cardiovascular Health:** The risk of heart disease and related conditions increases with age. Regular heart health assessments and preventive measures become even more crucial.

- **Prostate Health:** Prostate issues, including benign

prostatic hyperplasia (BPH) and prostate cancer, become more common. Monitoring and treatment options may be discussed.

- **Bone Health:** Osteoporosis can affect men in their senior years, making bone health maintenance essential.

- **Cognitive Health:** Age-related cognitive decline may occur. Engaging in mentally stimulating activities and maintaining social connections can support cognitive health.

- **Chronic Conditions:** Chronic conditions such as diabetes, hypertension, and arthritis may require ongoing management.

- **End-of-Life Planning:** Discussions about end-of-life

care preferences, living arrangements, and financial planning may become important.

- **Social Connections:** Maintaining social connections and support networks is vital for emotional well-being and resilience in later life.

Throughout all stages of life, regular health check-ups, preventive measures, and a proactive approach to health are essential. Consulting with healthcare providers and specialists as needed can help address age-related health concerns and optimize men's health and quality of life at every stage.

CHAPTER 5

Screening and Early Detection

Screening for various health conditions is a critical aspect of preventive healthcare. It involves the systematic assessment of individuals who may be at risk for certain diseases or conditions, even in the absence of symptoms. Early detection through screening can lead to timely interventions and improved outcomes. Here's an overview of the importance of screening, recommended screenings for men, and understanding test results:

5.1 The Importance of Screening

- **Early Detection:** Screening tests can identify health issues at an early stage, often before symptoms develop. Early detection allows for timely treatment and better chances of recovery.

- **Preventive Measures:** Many screenings help assess risk factors and allow individuals to take preventive measures to reduce the risk of developing certain conditions.

- **Improved Outcomes:** When health conditions are identified and treated early, the chances of successful treatment and recovery are generally higher.

- **Quality of Life:** Detecting and managing chronic conditions early can help improve one's overall quality of life by preventing complications and reducing the severity of the disease.

- **Cost-Effective:** Preventive screenings can be cost-effective in the long run by reducing the need for more expensive treatments and hospitalizations.

5.2 Recommended Screenings for Men

The specific screenings and recommended frequencies may vary based on age, family history, and individual risk factors. Men should discuss their screening needs with a healthcare provider, who can provide personalized recommendations. However, here are some common screenings for men:

- **Blood Pressure Measurement:** Regular blood pressure checks are crucial to monitor for hypertension, a risk factor for heart disease and stroke.

- **Cholesterol Testing:** This assesses levels of LDL ("bad") cholesterol and HDL ("good") cholesterol, which are related to heart health. High cholesterol is a risk factor for heart disease.

- **Blood Glucose Testing:** To screen for diabetes or prediabetes, especially if there are risk factors like obesity or a family history of diabetes.

- **Prostate-Specific Antigen (PSA) Test:** For prostate cancer screening, though its use and frequency are a subject of discussion due to potential overdiagnosis and overtreatment.

- **Colorectal Cancer Screening:** Methods include colonoscopy, sigmoidoscopy, and stool tests. The frequency and type of screening depend on age and risk factors.

- **Skin Cancer Screening:** Regular skin examinations, especially for individuals with a history of skin cancer or high sun exposure.

- **Bone Density Testing:** To assess bone health, particularly for older men at risk of osteoporosis.

- **Eye Exams:** Regular eye exams, especially for conditions like glaucoma and macular degeneration.

- **Dental Check-ups:** Regular dental visits for oral health assessments and preventive care.

- **Immunizations:** Vaccinations, including flu shots, pneumonia vaccines, and recommended booster shots.

- **Testicular Self-Exams:** Although not a formal screening, it's essential for men to be aware of their testicular health and report any changes to a healthcare provider.

5.3 Understanding Test Results

Understanding the results of screening tests is essential. Here are some key points:

- **Normal vs. Abnormal:** Tests often provide reference ranges that indicate what is considered normal. Abnormal results may suggest a health issue but do not necessarily confirm a diagnosis.

- **Follow-up:** If a test result is abnormal or indicates a potential problem, further evaluation or additional tests may be needed. Follow your healthcare provider's guidance.

- **Risk Factors:** Some screening results may be influenced by risk factors or other medical conditions. Discuss your results and any relevant factors with your healthcare provider.

- **Preventive Measures:** Regardless of the results, preventive measures like lifestyle changes, vaccinations, and regular check-ups are essential for maintaining good health.

- **Open Communication:** Maintain open and honest communication with your healthcare provider about your health concerns, family history, and any symptoms you may be experiencing.

- **Second Opinions:** If you have concerns about the interpretation of your test results or the recommended course of action, don't hesitate to seek a second opinion from another qualified healthcare provider.

regular screening and early detection of health conditions are vital for men's well-being. Understanding the importance of screening, staying informed about recommended screenings, and interpreting test results in consultation with healthcare providers can help men proactively manage their health and prevent or address potential health issues.

CHAPTER 6

Treatment and Management

Treatment and management of common men's health issues involve a combination of medical interventions, lifestyle modifications, and therapies aimed at improving overall well-being and addressing specific health conditions. In this section, we'll explore treatment options for common men's health issues and the role of medications and therapies:

6.1 Treatment Options for Common Men's Health Issues

Heart Health:

- Lifestyle Modifications: A heart-healthy lifestyle includes a balanced diet, regular exercise, smoking cessation, and stress management.

- Medications: Depending on the condition, medications such as statins, blood pressure drugs, and antiplatelet agents may be prescribed.

- Procedures: In some cases, procedures like angioplasty or bypass surgery may be necessary to address blocked arteries.

Prostate Health:

- Monitoring: For benign prostatic hyperplasia (BPH), watchful waiting or active surveillance may be recommended.

- Medications: Medications like alpha-blockers and 5-alpha reductase inhibitors can help manage BPH symptoms.

- Surgery: Surgical procedures like transurethral resection of the prostate (TURP) or laser therapy may be necessary for severe BPH.

- Prostate Cancer: Treatment options vary depending on the stage and aggressiveness of cancer and may include surgery, radiation therapy,

chemotherapy, hormone
therapy, or active surveillance.

Sexual Health:

- Erectile Dysfunction (ED):
  Treatment options include oral
  medications (e.g., Viagra),
  vacuum erection devices, penile
  injections, and surgery (penile
  implants).

- Low Testosterone: Hormone
  replacement therapy (HRT) can
  be prescribed to raise
  testosterone levels in cases of
  clinically low testosterone.

- Sexual Counseling: Mental
  health professionals or sexual
  health specialists can provide
  counseling and therapy for
  sexual issues.

Mental Health and Depression:

- Psychotherapy: Cognitive-behavioral therapy (CBT), interpersonal therapy, and other forms of counseling can help individuals manage depression.

- Medications: Antidepressant medications may be prescribed, such as selective serotonin reuptake inhibitors (SSRIs) or serotonin-norepinephrine reuptake inhibitors (SNRIs).

- Lifestyle Changes: Exercise, stress reduction, and social support are essential components of managing depression.

Substance Abuse and Addiction:

- Detoxification: In cases of addiction, medically supervised detoxification may be necessary to safely manage withdrawal symptoms.

- Rehabilitation Programs: Inpatient or outpatient rehabilitation programs offer structured support, counseling, and therapy to address addiction.

- Medication-Assisted Treatment (MAT): MAT combines counseling and behavioral therapy with medications (e.g., methadone, buprenorphine) to treat opioid addiction.

- Support Groups: Participating in support groups, such as Alcoholics Anonymous (AA) or Narcotics Anonymous (NA), can provide ongoing peer support.

6.2 Medications and Therapies

- **Medications:** Medications play a crucial role in the treatment of various men's health issues. For example, medications like statins, antihypertensives, and antiplatelet drugs are commonly used to manage heart disease. Erectile dysfunction can be treated with medications like sildenafil (Viagra). In the case of depression, antidepressants like sertraline (Zoloft) or therapy may be recommended. It's essential to follow prescribed medication regimens as directed by healthcare providers.

- **Therapies:** Therapies are valuable in addressing mental health concerns, including depression and addiction. Cognitive-behavioral therapy (CBT), talk therapy, psychoanalysis, and group therapy can be effective in treating mental health conditions. Behavioral therapies, such as contingency management or motivational enhancement therapy, are used in addiction treatment to modify behaviors and build coping skills.

- **Surgery and Procedures:** Surgical interventions may be necessary for certain conditions. For example, heart procedures like angioplasty or coronary artery bypass grafting (CABG) are performed to treat heart disease. Surgical options like prostatectomy are used in the management of prostate cancer.

- **Lifestyle Modifications:** Lifestyle changes, such as dietary improvements, regular exercise, smoking cessation, and stress management, are fundamental components of treatment and disease management for various men's health issues, including heart disease, prostate health, and mental health conditions.

- **Physical Therapy:** Physical therapy may be recommended for men recovering from surgery or injury, as well as for managing chronic pain or musculoskeletal conditions.

Treatment and management plans should be individualized based on a person's specific health condition, medical history, and preferences. It's crucial for men to work closely with their healthcare providers to develop and follow appropriate treatment plans, and to make necessary adjustments as needed to optimize their health and well-being.

6.3 Lifestyle Modifications

Lifestyle modifications are a cornerstone of preventive healthcare and can significantly impact men's health by reducing the risk of various conditions and improving overall well-being. Here are key lifestyle modifications for men to consider:

Diet and Nutrition:

- Adopt a balanced diet rich in fruits, vegetables, whole grains, lean proteins, and healthy fats.

- Limit saturated fats, trans fats, sodium, and added sugars.

- Control portion sizes to manage calorie intake.

- Stay hydrated by drinking plenty of water.

Physical Activity:

- Aim for at least 150 minutes of moderate-intensity aerobic exercise or 75 minutes of vigorous-intensity aerobic exercise per week, as recommended by guidelines.

- Incorporate strength training exercises at least two days a week to maintain muscle mass.

- Stay active throughout the day by reducing sedentary behavior.

Smoking Cessation:

- Quit smoking and avoid exposure to secondhand smoke. Smoking is a leading cause of preventable diseases, including heart disease and lung cancer.

Alcohol Moderation:

- If you choose to drink alcohol, do so in moderation. Guidelines suggest up to one drink per day for men.

- Be aware of the risks of excessive alcohol consumption, which can lead to liver disease, addiction, and accidents.

Stress Management:

- Practice stress-reduction techniques such as mindfulness, meditation, deep breathing exercises, and relaxation strategies.

- Develop healthy coping mechanisms for managing life's challenges.

Sleep Hygiene:

- Aim for 7-9 hours of quality sleep per night to support physical and mental health.

- Maintain a consistent sleep schedule and create a comfortable sleep environment.

Weight Management:

- Achieve and maintain a healthy
  weight through a combination
  of diet and exercise.

- Monitor caloric intake and be
  mindful of portion sizes.

Regular Health Check-ups:

- Schedule regular health check-
  ups with a healthcare provider
  to monitor blood pressure,
  cholesterol levels, and other
  vital signs.

- Follow recommended
  screenings and vaccinations
  based on age and risk factors.

Mental Health Care:

- Prioritize mental health by
  seeking support and therapy
  when needed.

- Foster social connections and maintain open communication with loved ones.

Substance Abuse Prevention:

- Avoid or quit substance abuse, including tobacco and illicit drugs.

- Seek help and support for addiction if necessary.

6.4 Surgery and Interventions

In some cases, medical interventions and surgical procedures may be necessary to treat or manage certain men's health conditions. Here are some examples:

Heart Health:

- Angioplasty: A procedure to open blocked or narrowed arteries using a small balloon and, in some cases, stent placement.

- Coronary Artery Bypass Grafting (CABG): Surgery to bypass blocked coronary arteries using blood vessels from another part of the body.

Prostate Health:

- Prostatectomy: Surgical removal of the prostate gland, often used in the treatment of prostate cancer.

- Transurethral Resection of the Prostate (TURP): A surgical procedure to treat benign prostatic hyperplasia (BPH) by removing excess prostate tissue.

Orthopedic Procedures:

- Joint Replacement: Surgical replacement of damaged joints, such as hips or knees, to alleviate pain and improve mobility.

- Arthroscopy: Minimally invasive surgical procedures to diagnose and treat joint conditions.

Cancer Treatment:

- Surgery may be a part of cancer treatment to remove tumors or affected tissue.

- Radiation therapy, chemotherapy, immunotherapy, and targeted therapy are also used in cancer treatment.

Reproductive Health:

- Vasectomy: A surgical procedure for permanent contraception by cutting or sealing the vas deferens.

- Fertility Treatments: Procedures like in vitro fertilization (IVF) or intracytoplasmic sperm injection (ICSI) may be used to address fertility issues.

Mental Health:

- Electroconvulsive Therapy (ECT): A treatment option for severe depression or other mental health conditions.

- Deep Brain Stimulation (DBS): Used for conditions like Parkinson's disease or treatment-resistant depression.

Urological Procedures:

- Urological surgeries may be performed for conditions such as kidney stones, urinary incontinence, or bladder issues.

The decision to undergo surgery or medical interventions is made in consultation with healthcare providers and specialists and is based on individual health conditions, risks, and potential benefits. It's essential for men to discuss their options, ask questions, and weigh the pros and cons before proceeding with any surgical or interventional treatments.

CHAPTER 7

Lifestyle and Wellness

Maintaining a healthy lifestyle is crucial for men's overall well-being and longevity. In this section, we'll explore tips for a healthy lifestyle, exercise and fitness routines, diet and nutrition guidelines, stress reduction techniques, and the importance of sleep and rest:

7.1 Tips for a Healthy Lifestyle

- **Stay Active:** Incorporate regular physical activity into your routine. Aim for a mix of

aerobic exercise, strength
training, and flexibility
exercises.

- **Balanced Diet:** Eat a balanced
diet rich in fruits, vegetables,
whole grains, lean proteins, and
healthy fats. Limit processed
foods, sugary beverages, and
excessive sodium.

- **Hydration:** Drink plenty of
water throughout the day to
stay hydrated. Limit sugary
drinks and excessive caffeine.

- **Moderate Alcohol:** If you
consume alcohol, do so in
moderation. Limit your intake
to recommended guidelines.

- **Tobacco-Free:** Avoid smoking
and exposure to secondhand
smoke. Seek support and

resources to quit if you're a smoker.

- **Regular Health Check-ups:** Schedule regular check-ups with a healthcare provider for preventive screenings and to monitor your health.

- **Mental Health Care:** Prioritize your mental health. Seek support and therapy when needed, and develop healthy coping mechanisms.

- **Healthy Relationships:** Cultivate healthy, supportive relationships with friends and family. Open communication and emotional intimacy are vital.

- **Stress Management:** Practice stress reduction techniques, such as mindfulness, meditation, deep breathing exercises, or hobbies you enjoy.

- **Adequate Sleep:** Aim for 7-9 hours of quality sleep per night by establishing a consistent sleep schedule and creating a comfortable sleep environment.

- **Safety:** Prioritize safety, whether it's on the road, at work, or during recreational activities. Wear protective gear when necessary.

7.2 Exercise and Fitness Routines

- **Aerobic Exercise:** Engage in aerobic activities like walking, jogging, swimming, cycling, or dancing for at least 150 minutes per week.

- **Strength Training:**
  Incorporate strength training
  exercises for all major muscle
  groups at least two days a
  week. This helps maintain
  muscle mass and bone density.

- **Flexibility and Balance:**
  Include stretching and balance
  exercises in your routine to
  improve flexibility and prevent
  injuries.

- **Variety:** Change up your
  exercise routine to prevent
  boredom and overuse injuries.
  Try new activities or classes to
  keep it interesting.

- **Consistency:** Make exercise a
  regular part of your routine by
  scheduling it, just like any other
  commitment.

7.3 Diet and Nutrition Guidelines

- **Fruits and Vegetables:** Aim for a variety of colorful fruits and vegetables, which provide essential vitamins and antioxidants.

- **Whole Grains:** Choose whole grains like brown rice, quinoa, whole wheat bread, and oats over refined grains.

- **Lean Proteins:** Include sources of lean protein, such as poultry, fish, beans, legumes, and tofu, in your diet.

- **Healthy Fats:** Opt for healthy fats found in avocados, nuts, seeds, and olive oil while limiting saturated and trans fats.

- **Portion Control:** Be mindful of portion sizes to prevent overeating.

- **Hydration:** Drink water regularly throughout the day and limit sugary beverages.

- **Limit Processed Foods:** Reduce your intake of highly processed foods, which often contain excess sodium, sugar, and unhealthy fats.

- **Moderate Alcohol:** If you consume alcohol, do so in moderation according to recommended guidelines.

7.4 Stress Reduction Techniques

- **Mindfulness Meditation:** Practice mindfulness to stay present and reduce stress.

- **Deep Breathing:** Incorporate deep breathing exercises to calm your nervous system.

- **Physical Activity:** Regular exercise is an effective stress reducer.

- **Hobbies and Leisure:** Engage in hobbies and activities you enjoy to unwind and relax.

- **Social Support:** Lean on friends and family for emotional support during stressful times.

- **Time Management:** Prioritize tasks, set realistic goals, and manage your time effectively.

7.5 Sleep and Rest

- **Sleep Routine:** Establish a consistent sleep schedule by going to bed and waking up at the same times each day, even on weekends.

- **Sleep Environment:** Create a comfortable sleep environment with a cool, dark, and quiet room.

- **Limit Screen Time:** Reduce exposure to screens (phones, tablets, computers) before bedtime to improve sleep quality.

- **Relaxation Techniques:** Engage in relaxing activities before bedtime, such as reading, gentle stretching, or taking a warm bath.

- **Caffeine and Alcohol:** Avoid excessive caffeine and alcohol consumption in the hours leading up to bedtime.

Prioritizing a healthy lifestyle, including exercise, nutrition, stress management, and adequate sleep, can have a profound impact on men's physical and mental well-being. Making small, sustainable changes over time can lead to significant improvements in overall health and quality of life.